# BTEC

## HEALTH AND SOCIAL CARE

### ASSESSMENT GUIDE

Level 2

## Unit 8 INDIVIDUAL RIGHTS IN HEALTH AND SOCIAL CARE

ELIZABETH RASHEED

HODDER
EDUCATION
AN HACHETTE UK COMPANY

The sample learner answers provided in this assessment guide are intended to give guidance on how a learner might approach generating evidence for each assessment criterion. Answers do not necessarily include all of the evidence required to meet each assessment criterion. Assessor comments intend to highlight how sample answers might be improved to help learners meet the requirements of the grading criterion but are provided as a guide only. Sample answers and assessor guidance have not been verified by Edexcel and any information provided in this guide should not replace your own internal verification process.

Any work submitted as evidence for assessment for this unit must be the learner's own. Submitting as evidence, in whole or in part, any material taken from this guide will be regarded as plagiarism. Hodder Education accepts no responsibility for learners plagiarising work from this guide that does or does not meet the assessment criteria.

The sample assignment briefs are provided as a guide to how you might assess the evidence required for all or part of the internal assessment of this unit. They have not been verified or endorsed by Edexcel and should be internally verified through your own Lead Internal Verifier as with any other assignment briefs, and/or checked through the BTEC assignment checking service.

Orders: please contact Bookpoint Ltd, 130 Milton Park, Telephone: +44 (0)1235 827720. Fax: +44 (0)1235 400454. Lines are open from 9.00 a.m. to 5.00 p.m., Monday to Saturday, with a 24-hour message answering service. You can also order through our website www.hoddereducation.co.uk

If you have any comments to make about this, or any of our other titles, please send them to educationenquiries@hodder.co.uk

*British Library Cataloguing in Publication Data*

A catalogue record for this title is available from the British Library

ISBN: 978 1 444 189865

Published 2013

Impression number    10 9 8 7 6 5 4 3 2 1

Year                       2016 2015 2014 2013

Copyright © 2013 Elizabeth Rasheed

Cover photo © vege – Fotolia.com

Typeset by Integra Software Services Pvt, Ltd., Pondicherry, India

Printed in Dubai for Hodder Education,
an Hachette UK Company,
338 Euston Road,
London NW1 3BH

# Contents

## For attention of the learner

You are not allowed to copy any information from this book and use it as your own evidence. That would count as plagiarism, which is taken very seriously and may result in disqualification. If you are in any doubt at all please speak to your teacher.

# Acknowledgments

## Photo credits

The authors and publishers would like to thank the following for the use of photographs in this volume:

Figure 1.1 © lawcain – Fotolia.com; Figure 1.2 © John Birdsall / Photofusion; Figure 1.3 © Sandor Kacso – Fotolia.com; Figure 2.1 © Alex Stojanov / Alamy; Figure 2.2 © OJO Images Ltd / Alamy; Figure 2.3 © Simone van den Berg – Fotolia.com

Every effort has been made to trace and acknowledge ownership of copyright. The publishers will be glad to make suitable arrangements with any copyright holders whom it has not been possible to contact.

# Command words

You will find the following command words in the assessment criteria for each unit.

| | |
|---|---|
| Analyse | Identify the factors that apply and state how these are related. Explain the importance of each one. |
| Assess | Give careful consideration to all the factors or events that apply and identify which are the most important or relevant. |
| Describe | Give a clear description that includes all the relevant features – think of it as 'painting a picture with words'. |
| Discuss | Consider different aspects of a topic and how they interrelate, and the extent to which they are important. |
| Evaluate | Bring together all the information and review it to form a conclusion. Give evidence for each of your views or statements. |
| Explain | Provide details and give reasons and/or evidence to support the arguments being made. Start by introducing the topic then give the 'how' or 'why'. |
| Summarise | Demonstrate an understanding of the key facts, and if possible illustrate with relevant examples. |
| Justify | Give reasons or evidence to support your opinion or veiws to show how you arrived at these conclusions. |

# UNIT 8
# Equality and Diversity in Health and Social Care

*Unit 8: Individual Rights in Health and Social Care* is an internally assessed, optional, specialist unit with two learning aims:

- **Learning aim A:** Investigate the rights of individuals using health and social care services.
- **Learning aim B:** Examine the responsibilities of employers and employees in upholding service users' rights in health and social care.

The unit focuses on the rights of people who use health and social care, including the right to be respected, to be treated equally and fairly, and not to be discriminated against. It also looks at how employers and employees in health and social care have a responsibility to make sure service users get their rights.

Learning aim A looks at the rights individuals have when they use health and social care services.

Learning aim B looks at the duty that employers and employees have to ensure that service users' rights are upheld and how this affects the people who use the services.

Each learning aim is divided into two sections. The first section focuses on the content of the learning aim and each of the topics is covered. At the end of each section there are knowledge recap questions to test your understanding of the subject. The answers for the knowledge recap questions can be found at the end of the guide.

The second section of each learning aim provides support with assessment by using evidence generated by a learner, for each grading criterion, with feedback from an assessor. The assessor has highlighted where the evidence is sufficient to satisfy the grading criterion and provided developmental feedback when additional work is required.

At the end of the guide are examples of assignment briefs for this unit. There is a sample assignment for each learning aim, and the tasks allow you to generate the evidence needed to meet all the assessment criteria in the unit.

# Learning aim A

## Investigate the rights of individuals using health and social care services

### Assessment criteria

**2A.P1** Summarise the individual rights of service users in health and social care.

**2A.P2** Describe how current and relevant legislation protects the rights of service users, using examples.

**2A.M1** Explain ways in which service users' individual rights can be upheld in health and social care, using selected examples.

**2A.D1** Assess the benefits and potential difficulties of upholding service users' rights in health and social care, using selected examples.

## The rights of individuals using health and social care services

Rights are what we are entitled to. We all have the following rights:

- **To be respected.** Mary has learning difficulties, lives in sheltered accommodation and is planning a holiday. She decides where she wants to go on holiday. The care workers do not make the decision for her. Her views are respected.
- **To be treated as an individual.** Javed is overweight and needs to manage his diet. He is vegetarian. The dietician should treat him as an individual and not make him adopt a non-vegetarian diet.
- **To be treated with dignity.** Douglas lives alone and has problems managing personal hygiene since his stroke left him paralysed on one side of his body. Dave, his carer, helps him to have a shower but also helps Douglas to do what he can for himself. Dave puts soap on the flannel but then Douglas can wash himself and maintain his dignity.
- **To be treated equally and not discriminated against.** Sam and Toni are a lesbian couple. Sam has to go into hospital for an operation and only next of kin are allowed to visit. Toni is allowed to visit as she is the civil partner. This is an example of treating people equally.

- **To be allowed privacy and confidentiality.** Zara goes to the surgery to make an appointment with her GP. The receptionist asks what the problem is. Zara feels she should not have to tell the receptionist private information and she complains to the surgery manager. The system is changed so that patients do not have to disclose confidential information at the reception desk. This change allows privacy and confidentiality for patients.

- **To be allowed access to information about self.** Saif has complex health needs. He is worried that his GP is not taking his health needs seriously. According to the NHS website:

  'If you want to view your health records, you may not need to make a formal application. Nothing in the law prevents healthcare professionals from informally showing you your own records. You can make an informal request during a consultation, or by phoning your GP surgery or hospital to arrange a time to see your records.'

- **To have account taken of own choices, for example to communicate in preferred method or language.** Chantelle is deaf from birth. She uses British Sign Language (BSL) to communicate. When she needs to go into hospital the NHS provides a signer so that Chantelle can communicate in her own language.

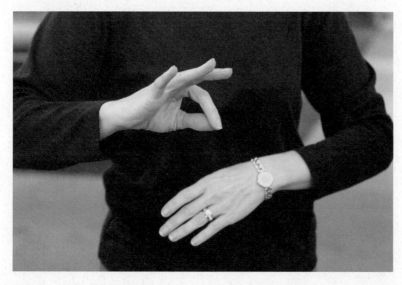

Figure 1.1 Everyone has the right to communicate in their own language

- **To be allowed independence.** May is going into a residential care home for the first time. She wants to stay as independent as possible and after discussion with the care manager she decides to manage her own medication.
- **To be safe.** Violet is 75 years old and lives at Poppydene Care Home. She has dementia and came into care because when living at home she would often go out and forget how to get back. In order to keep her safe at Poppydene, the carers make sure the front door is locked but Violet can go out in the garden, where she can be safely supervised.
- **To be able to take risks.** May is happy in the care home but wants to keep her independence. She takes the bus and meets friends once a week for coffee in town. May decides she can manage the risk and as a result she is able to stay independent.
- **To be involved in own care.** May, Chantelle, Sam and Douglas are involved in their own care. They are more likely to understand what they need to do and in this way they will remain healthier.

# Current and relevant legislation and how it protects the rights of service users

## Human Rights Act 1998

The **Human Rights Act 1998** states that your human rights are:

1. The right to life
2. Freedom from torture and degrading treatment
3. Freedom from slavery and forced labour
4. The right to liberty
5. The right to a fair trial
6. The right not to be punished for something that was not a crime when you did it
7. The right to respect for private and family life
8. Freedom of thought, conscience and religion, and freedom to express your beliefs
9. Freedom of expression
10. Freedom of assembly and association
11. The right to marry and to start a family
12. The right not to be discriminated against in respect of these rights and freedoms
13. The right to peaceful enjoyment of your property
14. The right to an education
15. The right to participate in free elections
16. The right not to be subjected to the death penalty.

If any one of these rights and freedoms is breached, you have a right to take the person to court, even if the breach was by someone in authority, such as a police officer.

## Equality Act 2010

The **Equality Act 2010** protects the rights of people who use health and social care services. It protects them from discrimination, harassment and victimisation on the grounds of age, disability, gender reassignment, marriage and civil partnership, pregnancy and maternity, race, religion or belief, sex and sexual orientation.

# Mental Health Act 1983

The **Mental Health Act 1983** and parts of the Mental Capacity Act 2005 were amended by the Mental Health Act 2007 which defined mental disorder as 'any disorder or disability of the mind'. To prevent discrimination and protect people, this definition cannot be used against people with learning disabilities unless that disability is 'associated with abnormally aggressive or seriously irresponsible conduct'.

Guiding principles in the Act include:

- **Purpose principle.** Decisions must be taken with the purpose of maximising the safety and wellbeing (mental and physical) of patients, promoting their recovery and protecting other people from harm.
- **Least restriction principle.** People taking action without a patient's consent must minimise the restrictions they impose on the patient's liberty.
- **Respect principle.** The diverse needs, values and circumstances of each patient must be respected, including their race, religion, culture, gender, age, sexual orientation and any disability.
- **Participation principle.** Patients must be involved in planning and reviewing their own treatment where possible.
- **Effectiveness, efficiency and equity.** People taking decisions under the Act must use resources in the most effective, efficient and equitable way.

The 2007 Act ensures patients are involved in their own care and that independent mental health advocacy is there to support patients. Patients have a right to refuse certain treatment such as electroconvulsive therapy (ECT). Some people with mental health issues realise they are unwell and volunteer to go into hospital. Others are forcibly detained, which conflicts with the right to liberty. Part of the 2007 Act is about the Deprivation of Liberty Safeguards (DoLS) which ensures that the right to liberty is respected where possible.

# How care workers can uphold the rights of service users

People who work in care should uphold service users' rights. This can at times be difficult but it is important to do so because of the benefits for service users. Here are some examples of how in health and social care settings, the rights of service users can be upheld and the difficulties and benefits of doing this.

## Anti-discriminatory practices

Studied

An activities coordinator for a care home planned a trip that included everyone, whatever their mobility issues, so that people using wheelchairs could also attend. It was not easy to find a coach that could take wheelchairs and it is often more expensive but eventually one was found. The benefit was that everyone was able to attend the trip, no one felt left out and it helped the residents bond as friends.

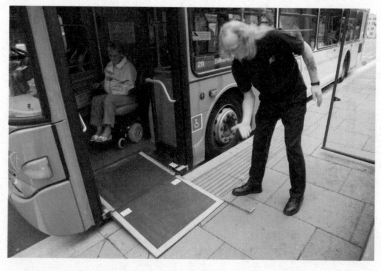

**Figure 1.2** Wheelchair accessible transport can help to ensure no one is discriminated against

## Ensuring privacy during personal care

Studied

Mr Zaid has dementia which means that he does not always communicate his need to use the toilet in time. He is incontinent. The carers take him to his room where in the privacy of his own bathroom he can be helped to have a shower and change his clothes. It is difficult to care for someone who wets or soils themselves, especially when that person is not fully aware of what is happening. Carers might feel disgust, and other residents may not be sympathetic; nevertheless a carer must put aside any personal feelings they have and must treat Mr Zaid with care and compassion. The benefit of this is that he is treated with respect and his dignity is ensured. A further benefit is that other residents seeing him treated with dignity will know that if they are ever in that situation they too will be treated with respect.

## Offering a person-centred approach

Mrs Khan, a resident in a care home, is diabetic and likes an early morning shower. The manager involves Mrs Khan in her own care by negotiating a safe time for her shower. Together they assess the risks of a home visit and the impact on Mrs Khan's routine. Mrs Khan likes to keep control of her diabetes herself, does her own blood sugar tests and manages her insulin with the help of the nurse. This person-centred approach means she can go out with relatives and independently decide when she has her meal and insulin. A person-centred approach gives choice. Mrs Khan's case study shows person-centred care in practice.

One difficulty with offering person-centred care is that carers have less control. Clients may take risks. Many carers worry that they may be blamed for poor care if anything goes wrong and so try to reduce risk by controlling every aspect of care and denying the client choice. Changing attitudes among carers is one major difficulty in offering person-centred care.

Another difficulty is that person-centred care takes time. A carer has to know the service user's capacity for independence. Person-centred care must be tailored for the individual, so although it may be safe for Mrs Khan to go out, it might not be safe for someone with dementia.

The benefits of person-centred care are life changing for service users. Being able to make their own decisions means they continue hobbies or employment, stay independent and be healthier for longer. They have a greater sense of wellbeing and require less care.

# Showing empathy

Mr Zaid has dementia and at times undresses in the sitting room of the care home, thinking it is his own home. He is treated with dignity and respect, and led to his own room when this happens. Carers show empathy. They try to put themselves in Mr Zaid's situation and think what he would prefer. At times, other residents complain about his behaviour and ask what is wrong with him and why he does it. The carers understand the right to privacy and confidentiality, so explain that Mr Zaid is not well. They do not tell the other residents that he has dementia. They empathise with him and his condition, maintain confidentiality and respect him as an individual, even though at times he is verbally abusive to them.

It is difficult at times to show empathy to someone who is abusive, but the carers know that Mr Zaid may not be aware of what he is saying, and he may be feeling frightened, humiliated and frustrated that he cannot remember. They know from their training not to take it personally but to step back, give him space and try to reassure him calmly when he swears at them. They also looked for triggers for the abuse and realised that he swears when he has wet himself. Realising this they now see when he is beginning to get agitated and ask if he wants the toilet. This has reduced the number of abusive incidents and also the number of times he is incontinent.

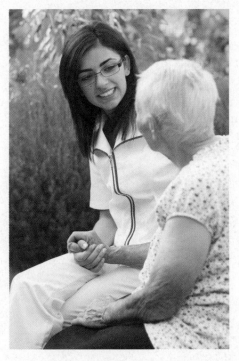

**Figure 1.3** It is important to empathise with a patient, understanding why they might behave in a certain way

Learning aim A: Investigate the rights of individuals using health and social care services

Showing empathy like this is difficult. It takes time, patience and a willingness to do the best for the person. The benefits are enormous. Mr Zaid has a better quality of life and better care because his carers show empathy. He is less aggressive which makes life easier for himself, the carers and other residents in the home.

## Being honest

Studied ▢

Being honest is very important. Honesty such as not stealing is of course essential and criminal record checks are carried out on all care workers, as no one would want to be cared for by someone they cannot trust. That type of honesty is vital. Telling the truth is also important, but care workers should know when to be totally open and when to wait before giving information.

Mrs Burton used to be the headteacher of a local school and is very alert. Following sudden weight loss she is admitted to hospital. Several tests are done. Staff nurse Jenny sees the results, as Mrs Burton is her patient, and she sees the suggested diagnosis but waits until the doctor is available to speak to Mrs Burton. He comes to discuss the results with Mrs Burton. Nurse Jenny is there to support her.

The doctor is very honest with Mrs Burton. The results show that she has advanced cancer of the stomach. There are several options for what to do next, but because the cancer has spread the treatments cannot cure her. Nurse Jenny knew the results indicated this but waited until the doctor had told Mrs Burton, because it is the doctor's job to give the diagnosis. The nurse's job is to help the patient understand what the doctor has said.

Being honest with a patient is important, but it takes a great deal of skill and it is difficult to know when to speak out and when to keep quiet. It is also emotionally very demanding. Another difficulty is that it requires training so that carers know what rights their patients have.

The benefits do, however, outweigh the difficulties. An honest care professional will inspire trust. Mrs Burton respected the doctor and the nurse for being honest with her. Although it was bad news, she knew the reality of the situation and had time to make her will, to arrange her funeral and see her family and friends before she died.

## Knowledge recap questions

1.  Name eleven rights of individuals using health and social care services.

2.  Give three examples of legislation that protect the rights of service users.

3.  Name five ways that care workers can uphold the rights of service users.

# Assessment guidance for Learning aim A

## Scenario

Your work placement has been arranged at a care home. Before starting, you want to make sure you know the rights of service users and what staff should do to make sure those rights are given.

Research the topics and make yourself a handbook to include the following sections:

*Individual rights of care service users, including current and relevant legislation*

Give a summary of the individual rights of care service users, referring to current and relevant legislation where appropriate.

*The responsibilities of care staff in dealing with service users*

Include a detailed explanation, using three examples, of ways in which the rights of service users can be upheld in care centres.

Give an assessment of the benefits to service users of having their rights upheld and any difficulties this may create for care staff.

### 2A.P1 Summarise the individual rights of service users in health and social care

**Assessor report:** The command verb in the grading criteria is **summarise**. In the learner's answer we would expect to see a short review of all the individual rights, with each one related to health and social care. The rights are to be respected, treated as an individual, treated with dignity, treated equally and not discriminated against, to be allowed privacy and confidentiality, access to information about self, to have account taken of their own choices, to be allowed independence, to be safe, able to take risks and to be involved in their own care.

## ✍ Learner answer

People who use health and social care services have these rights:

- to be respected – to be appreciated for who you are
- to be treated as an individual, not stereotyped as part of a group
- to be treated with dignity and not made fun of
- to be treated equally and not discriminated against so each person has the same chances
- to be allowed privacy, one's own space, and confidentiality so that private information is not given to those who do not have right to it
- to be allowed access to information about self so you can see what is written about you and have it corrected if it is wrong
- to have account taken of own choices, e.g. to communicate in preferred method or language so that other people do not make decisions for you
- to be allowed independence so that you have freedom to make your own decisions.

**Assessor report:** The learner has listed each of the individual rights of service users. They now need to summarise these rights, relating each one to health and social care.

## ✍ Learner answer

Jamie is 12 and has been taken into care because his parents cannot care for him as they are both addicted to heroin. He has a right to be treated as an individual. He goes to St Michael's School and on Tuesday evenings goes to karate classes.

He has the right to be respected **(a)**. He is very worried about his parents and about what will happen to them and to him. The social worker in charge of his case spends time with him and listens to his concerns, showing she respects him.

He has the right to be treated as an individual **(a)**, so she ensures he continues at the same school and can attend karate classes. She does not patronise him or tell him what to do, but treats him with dignity, and sets out the options available for his future. He can stay at the residential children's home and then go into foster care with a family until his own parents are able to care for him.

Jamie is from a rough part of town, where crime and addiction rates are high. He has had to fend for himself for most of his life. His clothes are dirty and he is not used to sitting down for a meal with others at a table. Some of the other children in the home start to make fun of him, but the staff intervene and talk to them, explaining that they all have the right to be treated equally and not discriminated against.

Jamie has the right to privacy and confidentiality **(a)**. This means that only those who need to know, such as his parents, social worker and teacher, will know he is in care and the reasons for this. The students in his class do not need to know and will not be told unless he chooses to tell them.

He also has the right to see what is written about him and to be involved in his own care **(a)**. He asks the social worker if he can see his file. She shows him what has been written and he points out that they have not put down that he likes playing football so she adds a bit about his football.

He has the right to have account taken of his own choices **(a)**. The social worker arranged a meeting for him with a couple who want to foster. They came to see him at the home. He was a bit wary and told the social worker later that he did not really like them. She decided to arrange a meeting with another couple and this time Jamie really got on with them.

**Assessor report:** The learner has summarised some of the rights of individuals.

## Assessor report – overall

*What is good about this assessment evidence?*

The learner has summarised most of the rights of individuals and also applied these to a social care situation showing their understanding of how the rights work in practice **(a)**.

*What could be improved about this assessment evidence?*

To achieve 2A.P1, the remaining rights should be included. These are the right to be safe and to be able to take risks.

(2A.P2) **Describe how current and relevant legislation protects the rights of service users, using examples**

• • • • • • • • • • • • • • • • • • • • • • • • • • • •

**Assessor report:** The command verb in the grading criteria is **describe**. In the learner's answer we would expect to see current and relevant legislation, including a reference to the Equality Act 2010. The learner should describe at least two ways that legislation protects the rights of service users and could apply this to a group of service users such as patients in hospital or residents in a care home.

## ✍ Learner answer

The Equality Act 2010 protects people from discrimination, harassment and victimisation on the grounds of age, disability, gender reassignment, marriage and civil partnership, pregnancy and maternity, race, religion or belief, sex and sexual orientation.

Life can be difficult for gay, lesbian and transgender people in care homes. According to rights given in the Equality Act 2010, same-sex couples have the same rights as heterosexual couples when it comes to accommodation. If a heterosexual couple would be housed together then same-sex couples should also be. Many older gay or lesbian people face discrimination in care homes but the Equality Act 2010 has given them the right to challenge this discrimination **(a)**.

**Assessor report:** The learner has made a good start by introducing one of the main pieces of legislation on equality, the Equality Act 2010, and giving an example **(a)**.

## Assessor report – overall

*What is good about this assessment evidence?*

The learner gives the correct name for the Act, the date and describes how this Act protects people. The learner also gives an example of how this applies to residents in a care home.

*What could be improved about this assessment evidence?*

The learner should describe other laws such as the Human Rights Act 1998, and the Mental Health Act 1983 (amended 2007), and should give at least two examples to illustrate their answer.

## 2A.M1 Explain ways in which service users' individual rights can be upheld in health and social care, using selected examples

Assessor report: The command verb in the grading criteria is **explain**. In the learner's answer we would expect to see details of how to uphold service users' individual rights. A minimum of three detailed examples from a range of settings will be needed, showing in each example the ways rights can be upheld and the legislation that gives these rights.

### ✍ Learner answer

The rights of service users can be upheld through:

● anti-discriminatory practices
● ensuring privacy during personal care
● offering person-centred approach
● showing empathy
● being honest.

Assessor report: The learner has made a good start by listing the ways in which service users' individual rights can be upheld in health and social care. They now need to explain how these rights are upheld, using at least three detailed examples.

### ✍ Learner answer

Older people who are gay, lesbian or transgender have the same rights as heterosexual people under the Equality Act 2010. This means that care homes must not discriminate against them when it comes to admission policies. A care home cannot refuse to admit an older person on the grounds of their sexuality **(a)**.

They must have the same privacy as everyone else during personal care and they must be offered person-centred care which looks at their needs as an individual. They may wish to share a room with their partner and if the home offers rooms for couples, residents cannot be discriminated against because of their sexual orientation.

Anti-discriminatory practices include the way that staff treat residents, but also how residents treat each other. Some residents may refuse to sit next to a gay person in the dining room. The care home manager has a duty to prevent discrimination by staff, other residents or visitors by tackling such discrimination if it arises. Even if they personally believe that homosexuality is wrong, they must uphold the Equality Act 2010 and the Human Rights Act and prevent discrimination **(a)**.

Showing empathy does not necessarily mean agreeing with someone, but it does mean trying to understand them. Anti-discriminatory practices include person-centred care, so the needs of the resident are met wherever possible. The care manager may find it difficult to prevent discrimination from other residents and they should be honest with the gay resident so that other ways may be tried to develop tolerance if this is the case. The care manager has much more power in the way staff treat residents, and any member of staff who is discriminatory should be dealt with by retraining or if that fails, by being sacked.

The Human Rights Act 1998 gives the right to respect for private and family life and freedom to express your beliefs as well as the right not to be discriminated against in respect of these rights and freedoms **(a)**. Some residents may feel that by not being allowed to express their disapproval of homosexuality, their freedoms are being restricted. This is a difficult situation for a care manager as rights may conflict. Sometimes the care manager may have to focus on building bridges between different residents so they develop tolerance.

*A second example*

People who have learning disabilities may experience discrimination from members of the public and sometimes from health and social care professionals.

People with learning disabilities have the same rights as anyone else under the Human Rights Act and the Equality Act 2010 (a). The only time when they may need someone to act on their behalf is when they lack the capacity to make decisions for themselves.

Sometimes some health care professionals do not understand learning disabilities and do not know that when a person with learning disabilities goes into hospital they have a duty to make reasonable adjustments to the treatment they provide for them. Anti-discriminatory practices mean that information should be available for the patient in a way they can understand. Leaflets should have plain, straightforward language and a learning disabilities nurse should be available to make sure the patient understands what is happening.

People with learning disabilities are entitled to the same privacy as everyone else during personal care. A person-centred approach means that care professionals will plan care according to individual needs. Sometimes a person with learning disabilities may have a passport stating their needs especially if they find it difficult to express themselves.

Hospitals are busy and frightening places for all patients, but especially so for people with learning difficulties. For this reason the care professional should take time and try to understand the needs of the patient. They should be honest. If an injection is going to hurt they should explain that it will hurt but only for a short time. It could be that an alternative form of medication could be used. By having empathy, the care professional will do their best to uphold the rights of the person with learning disabilities and ensure they are given their rights under the Equality Act 2010 which protects people from discrimination on the grounds of disability (a).

**Assessor report:** The learner has made a good start in explaining the ways in which service users' individual rights can be upheld in health and social care.

## Assessor report – overall

*What is good about this assessment evidence?*

The learner has given two detailed examples showing how rights can be upheld in two different settings. They have linked to relevant legislation (a).

*What could be improved about this assessment evidence?*

To achieve 2A.M1, a third example is required. As yet the learner has not mentioned the Mental Health Act so this third example should incorporate it to ensure full coverage of the legislation.

## 2A.D1 Assess the benefits and potential difficulties of upholding service users' rights in health and social care, using selected examples

Assessor report: The command verb in the grading criteria is **assess**. In the learner's answer we would expect to see how they weigh up the benefits and potential difficulties of upholding service users' rights using examples. A good answer might look at the difficulties that occur when there is a conflict between an individual service user's rights and the rights of other service users or the responsibilities of staff.

### ✍ Learner answer

We have seen that older people who are gay, lesbian or transgender have the same rights as heterosexual people, under the Equality Act 2010 and that employers and employees in health and social care have a responsibility to make sure these rights are put into practice.

Difficulties arise when upholding service users' rights. When staff uphold the rights of gay people, heterosexual people may feel they are not valued and may resent what they see as favouritism. They may say that they do not wish to live in the same home as a gay person **(a)**.

There are other difficulties in upholding rights. Some carers and residents are not tolerant. Their attitude is a barrier to equal rights. Sometimes people have strong religious beliefs and think homosexuality is a sin. They express their prejudice loudly and can bully and harass a gay person so their visitors feel uncomfortable and the resident becomes isolated. That can make other residents feel scared and upset them. Visitors, other residents and staff may feel uncomfortable if they do not understand sexual issues and so they may avoid talking to a gay or lesbian resident, isolating them further. Bullying and harassment should never be tolerated but it can take a long time to change attitudes **(a)**.

Staff should treat each resident as an equal individual. The benefits of doing this are that everyone will know that staff treat all people with respect. Individuals will feel valued. Residents will know they can trust staff to treat them fairly too. Staff will also feel good because they know they are giving good care and visitors will know that bullying is not tolerated so will feel happier about leaving their relatives in the care home **(b)**.

**Assessor report:** The learner has made a good start in assessing the benefits **(b)** and potential difficulties **(a)** of upholding service users' rights in health and social care.

## Assessor report – overall

*What is good about this assessment evidence?*

The learner has examined difficulties and benefits for one example.

*What could be improved about this assessment evidence?*

It would be good to see a summing up and a decision on whether benefits outweigh difficulties. Two further examples are required to provide a range across health and social care. These could be developed from examples raised in 2A.M1.

# Learning aim B

Examine the responsibilities of employers and employees in upholding service users' rights in health and social care

## Assessment criteria

**2B.P3** Describe how an employee can plan to maximise the safety of service users.

**2B.M2** Explain why risk assessment is important in health and social care.

**2B.D2** Evaluate the importance of the use of risk assessments in health and social care, using selected examples.

**2B.P4** Describe how the right to confidentiality is protected in health and social care.

**2B.M3** Explain why the right to confidentiality is protected in health and social care, using examples.

**2B.D3** Justify occasions where there is a need for an employee to breach confidentiality, using examples.

## Responsibilities of employers and employees in ensuring safety

Employers and the people who work for them, the employees, must ensure the safety of service users. Ways of ensuring safety are explained in this section.

### Risk assessment

Studied ▢

This involves assessing risk in a health and social care setting, saying why it is important, and acknowledging the right to take acceptable risks. It is impossible to get rid of all risks but we can manage them and reduce their impact.

Assessing risk is a five-step process to examine the workplace and prevent or reduce the risk of harm:

## Step 1: Identify the hazards

A **hazard** is anything that may cause harm, such as loose carpet, wet floor or trailing cord. The **risk** is the chance, high or low, that somebody could be harmed by these and other hazards, together with an indication of how serious the harm could be.

Sue, the manager of Poppydene Care Home, spotted a temporary hazard. When the cleaner vacuumed the sitting room, the wire from the vacuum cleaner to the plug trailed across the hall, creating a hazard. There was a high risk of people tripping over it. Slips, trips and falls are the major cause of accidents.

## Step 2: Decide who might be harmed and how

Sue realised that the care workers, visitors, and residents were all people who might trip over the cable and have a nasty fall.

## Step 3: Evaluate the risks and decide on precautions

She realised the trailing cable posed a high risk, and there was a nearer socket that could reduce the risk posed by trailing cables. She explained the risks to the cleaner and that the nearer socket must be used to reduce risk.

## Step 4: Record your findings and implement them

Sue noted the incident, told the staff and then put up a notice telling the staff to use the nearest socket for electrical equipment so they would not forget. Her risk assessment recorded what the hazard was, whether it was high or low risk, and what might happen. She then noted what action was needed, what was done, by whom and when. Sue had to prioritise and deal with those hazards that were high risk and had serious consequences first. She then looked at other hazards and assessed the risks in the same way.

## Step 5: Review your assessment and update if necessary

Sue reviewed the risk assessment. One of the cleaners had been on holiday when Sue drew staff attention to the hazard, and later a new cleaner started working at the home, so Sue had to review the risk assessment again to make sure everyone was following safe practice.

The right to take acceptable risks is part of choice. Sue carried out a risk assessment when Mrs Khan's family wanted to take their mum out. The potential hazards were that Mrs Khan could eat the wrong foods and not take her insulin on time. After making sure that Mrs Khan and her relatives understood the importance of the right food and timing of insulin, Mrs Khan decided for herself that the risks were low. This was her choice.

Mr Zaid's family wanted to take him out but when the care manager explained how he sometimes behaved due to his dementia, they felt they could not manage if he became aggressive (the hazard) and the risk to others was high. Instead, they compromised by bringing his grandchildren to visit him in the home where carers were at hand if he became aggressive.

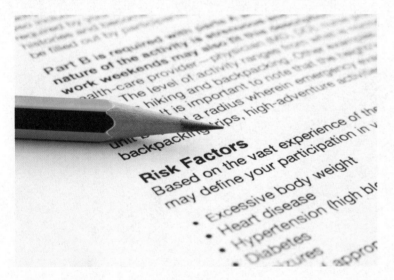

Figure 2.1 A risk assessment highlights any potential risks and how they might be reduced or managed

# Safeguarding – preventing harm

Safeguarding is part of the duty of care. It is important to prevent harm and carers have a duty to safeguard the individual, other residents, staff and themselves.

Mr Zaid's dementia means he gets confused and at times can be violent. The care manager has a duty to safeguard the other residents, the staff and Mr Zaid himself. She does this by risk assessing the situation.

She knows that when Mr Zaid wants the toilet he becomes agitated and because he is confused, he cannot express his needs. At these times he gets verbally abusive and can hit out at staff. Other residents get annoyed with him and have threatened him. The hazard of aggressive behaviour poses a high risk to everyone.

Sue asks staff to take Mr Zaid to the toilet every two hours to reduce the risk of his being incontinent, and reduce the risk of him becoming agitated and aggressive. This works up to a point but there are still times when he gets angry.

Sue reviews the situation and allocates Mr Zaid a main carer, Bill, who has had training in dementia care. Bill is able to understand Mr Zaid and his needs and to help others understand him. Bill finds out that Mr Zaid was a keen gardener and brings in seeds for him to plant. Gradually, Mr Zaid's frustration and anger are reduced and other residents are no longer angry with him.

# Other ways of ensuring safety

## Control of substances harmful to health

Ensuring safety is everyone's job. The **Control of Substances Hazardous to Health Regulations (COSHH)** is the law that says how employers must manage such substances as **chemicals**, **fumes**, **gases**, germs and body waste. Bleach and cleaning fluids must be stored in a locked cupboard and not put into other containers. The person who uses the bleach has a responsibility to lock it away. The manager has a responsibility to provide a place where it can be locked.

In health and social care settings all tablets and medication must be kept in a locked cupboard, which is secured to the wall. A record is kept of which medication is given when and by whom. Controlled drugs must be stored in a specially designed, double-locked cupboard and a strict record kept of what is used. Any medicines left over must be properly disposed of by the pharmacist. Only people trained to give medication may do so. Following these measures will ensure only the right drug in the right amount is given at the right time to the right person.

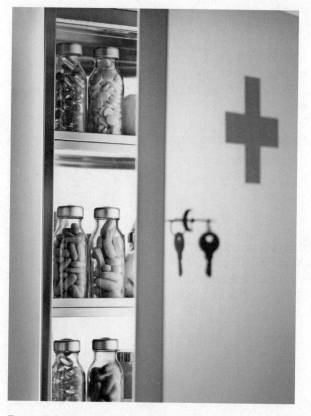

**Figure 2.2** Dangerous substances, such as chemicals and medicines, should be kept in a locked cupboard

## Use of protective equipment and infection control

Gloves and aprons must be provided by the employer. Employees must use them to reduce the risk of spreading infection. It is everyone's responsibility to control the spread of germs and one of the main ways to reduce the spread of infection is through hand-washing. Employers may have written procedures but it is the care workers' responsibility to wash their hands before and after care, and after going to the toilet. This prevents the spread of germs and reduces cross-infection.

## Reporting and recording accidents and incidents

This is again everyone's responsibility. Employees must report accidents and incidents. Each health and social care setting has a procedure for this, and has an accident or incident book. The person in charge may take a verbal report from people involved and complete the written report.

**Reporting of Injuries, Diseases and Dangerous Occurrences Regulations 1995 (RIDDOR)** says employers, the self-employed and people in control of work premises (the Responsible Person) must report certain serious workplace accidents, occupational diseases and near-misses to the Health and Safety Executive.

## Complaints procedures

Everyone in the care setting should know how to make a complaint. These procedures must be in place in a health and social care setting. A good care setting will act promptly and ensure complaints are dealt with as soon as possible.

## Provision of toilets, washing facilities and drinking water

This is an employer's responsibility. Staff should never share the toilets or washing facilities of service users.

## Provision of first aid facilities

The Health and Safety (First Aid) Regulations 1981 require all employers to provide adequate and appropriate first aid facilities. This is an employer's responsibility. There must be a trained first-aider. All staff should know where the first aid box is kept and who the trained first-aider is.

# Current and relevant legislation

The **Health and Safety at Work Act 1974** says that employers must:

- make the workplace safe, ensure machinery is safe and that safe systems of work are set and followed
- ensure articles and substances are moved, stored and used safely
- provide adequate welfare facilities
- train workers on health and safety
- consult workers on these matters.

**Reporting of Injuries, Diseases and Dangerous Occurrences Regulations 1995 (RIDDOR)** state that employers must report serious workplace accidents, occupational diseases and specified dangerous occurrences (near-misses).

The following regulations govern safe lifting:

- The Manual Handling Operations Regulations 1992 (amended 2002)
- Lifting Operations and Lifting Equipment Regulations 1998 (LOLER)
- Workplace, Health, Safety and Welfare Regulations 1992.

The **Control of Substances Hazardous to Health Regulations (COSHH) 2002** govern the storage of substances.

# Responsibilities of employers and employees in ensuring confidentiality

## Accurate recording and proper storage and retrieval of information

- This includes electronic methods, written records, the use of photographs, mobile phones and social media. Confidentiality or privacy of information relates to Article 8 of the European Convention of Human Rights. It extends to written and spoken information, as well as electronically held material.
- Information must be accurately recorded, stored safely and be retrievable.
- Written records must be factual, readable and signed and dated by the person making the record.
- Photographs may only be taken with permission and for relevant purposes; for example, to record injuries after an attack on a person. They may not be taken on personal equipment such as a camera phone, but must be taken by the official photographer using official equipment. Photographs form part of the medical record. Care professionals must maintain confidentiality.
- Using mobile phones to take photographs of patients and their relatives is unethical.
- Care workers must never discuss patients on social media such as Facebook, just as they are not allowed to discuss patients outside the work environment.

## Disclosure

This means giving information. Disclosure may refer to when a person discloses confidential information to a care professional. Disclosure may involve a care worker passing on information. According to the Nursing and Midwifery Council guidance, disclosure is only lawful and ethical if the individual has freely and fully given consent to the information being passed on. Consent may be explicit or implied. It may be required by law or be capable of justification by reason of the public interest, for example, if a patient tells a nurse they are going to kill someone or if a child tells a care worker that someone has sexually abused them.

# Maintaining confidentiality

This is important:

Studied

- to safeguard service users
- to adhere to legal and workplace requirements
- to respect the rights of service users.

Mrs X is a victim of domestic violence. She is discharged from hospital to a safe refuge. Her husband demands to know where she is. In a case like this, confidentiality must be maintained to protect Mrs X. Professional codes of conduct demand confidentiality and it is Mrs X's human right under the law.

## When breaches of confidentiality are appropriate

Occasionally, it may be necessary to breach confidentiality, for example:

- to safeguard other individual(s)
- to safeguard a service user
- to report criminal activities.

In such circumstances, protocol must be followed. Police do not automatically have the right to access information. Here is an example where a breach of confidentiality may be needed to safeguard an individual.

A child is admitted to hospital with recent injuries and injuries sustained over time. She says her aunt and aunt's boyfriend beat her. The professionals involved should raise concerns. This is an example of when it is appropriate to breach confidentiality.

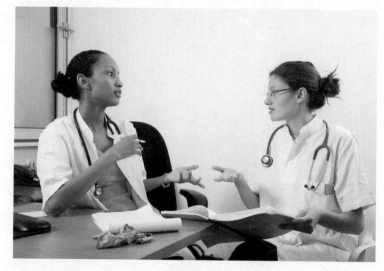

**Figure 2.3** There are instances where it is appropriate to breach patient confidentiality

Learning aim B: Examine the responsibilities of employers and employees

## Current and relevant legislation

The **Data Protection Act 1998** covers holding, obtaining, recording, using and disclosing of information that identifies living individuals. The Act applies to all forms of media, including paper and electronic.

The **Freedom of Information Act 2000**, which came into force in 2005, grants people rights of access to information not covered by the Data Protection Act 1998; for example, information which does not contain a person's identifiable details.

The **Police and Criminal Evidence Act 1984** allows nurses and midwives to pass on information to the police if they believe that someone may be seriously harmed, or death may occur if the police are not informed. There is a formal procedure that must be followed for this.

## Knowledge recap questions

1. Who must ensure the safety of service users?
2. Name the five steps in risk assessment.
3. What is the difference between a risk and a hazard?
4. When are breaches of confidentiality appropriate?
5. Give two examples of laws relating to confidentiality.

# Assessment guidance for Learning aim B

## Scenario

Your work placement has been arranged at a care home. Before starting you want to make sure you know the responsibilities of employers and employees in ensuring safety and confidentiality.

In the second part of your handbook include two sections: one about the responsibilities of care staff in ensuring safety, and the second section about the responsibilities of care staff in ensuring confidentiality for service users.

*The responsibilities of care staff in **ensuring safety for** service users*

In this section you will need:

- a detailed example, from a particular care setting, of how an employee can make sure care service users are safe
- an explanation of why the use of risk assessment is important for the wellbeing of service users in health and social care settings
- an evaluation, using two examples, of why it is important to carry out risk assessments in care settings.

*The responsibilities of care staff in **ensuring confidentiality for** service users*

Include the following:

- a description of how service user confidentiality is promoted in a particular care setting
- an explanation of why the right to confidentiality is important in care settings
- give two examples, from a care setting, of where a breach of confidentiality could be justified, explaining why breaking confidentiality is justified in each situation.

33

# Describe how an employee can plan to maximise the safety of service users

**Assessor report:** The command verb in the grading criteria is **describe**. In the learner's answer we would expect to see a description illustrating the main ways an employee can plan to maximise the safety of service users within a specific health and social care setting, through risk assessment, safeguarding, and other ways such as control of substances harmful to health, the use of protective equipment, infection control, reporting and recording accidents and incidents, dealing with complaints, the provision of staff toilets, washing facilities and drinking water, and the provision of first aid facilities.

## Learner answer

At Hazelwood Day Centre the staff ensure safety for service users in a variety of ways. The manager carries out a risk assessment using the five-step process:

1. Identify the hazards
2. Decide who might be harmed and how
3. Evaluate the risks and decide on precautions
4. Record your findings and implement them
5. Review your assessment and update if necessary.

She looks at the centre activities for service users in general but then does a risk assessment tailored to each individual's needs.

Mrs Jones cannot see and uses a white stick. The driver escorts her into the hall and hands over to day centre staff. The manager identifies the hazards such as chair legs sticking out, tables crowded together and bags on the floor. She evaluates the risks and decides there is a high risk of tripping, not just for Mrs Jones, but for everyone.

The manager records what she has found and decides to reduce the risk by making a rule that everyone should tuck their chair under the table when they get up. This does not get rid of the risk of tripping entirely but it reduces it.

Another rule is that all bags must be kept in lockers at the end of the room so no one can trip over them. This gets rid of the risk of tripping over bags.

She decides to rearrange the furniture, leaving a good space between tables so people can pass each other.

She implements these rules at the end of the morning, introducing them to staff and service users and explains why they are being brought in. She listens to their suggestions too. Someone suggest that when tea is being served, service users should sit down until everyone has their tea, to avoid bumping into a member of staff carrying a hot cup of tea. This will also prevent anyone slipping on spilled tea, as staff will have time to mop any spills before people get up. They all decide this is a good idea so add that to the list.

The manager monitors the situation for a month and is pleased to see there are no accidents and no near misses, which is an improvement on previous months. A new service user who uses a wheelchair is about to join the group, so the manager reviews the current risk assessment and updates it for a wheelchair user.

The manager takes her responsibilities seriously. Every new member of staff who starts has to have a police clearance check and other checks for working with vulnerable adults before they are allowed to start. Volunteers are never left alone with service users. All staff and volunteers have training on infection control and the use of protective equipment, such as gloves and aprons, in case of any blood or body fluid spills. They are trained on the safe storage of chemicals and control of substances harmful to health, such as bleach, which must be stored in a locked cupboard.

There is a staff toilet which is separate to that of service users and they have hand-washing facilities. All staff are trained how to manage complaints. They know to listen to the person and try to understand the problem, to offer the person a complaints form and pass that on to the manager.

**Assessor report:** The learner has made a good start in describing how an employee can plan to maximise the safety of service users.

## Assessor report – overall

*What is good about this assessment evidence?*

The learner has applied the information to a specific care setting and described the role of care managers and employees in ensuring safety. The learner has covered many of the ways of ensuring safety.

*What could be improved about this assessment evidence?*

In order to achieve 2B.P3, the learner should describe the reporting and recording of accidents and incidents and the provision of first aid facilities in this setting.

# Explain why risk assessment is important in health and social care

**Assessor report:** The command verb in the grading criteria is **explain**. In the learner's answer we would expect to see links to legislation such as the Health and Safety at Work Act 1974, and a detailed explanation of the importance of risk assessment in a specific health and social care setting. The learner should focus on a specific situation, for example risk assessing a trip to the local garden centre for residents of a care home, or a day trip to the seaside for those attending a day centre for people with learning disabilities. Learners who find it difficult to explain why risk assessment is important may be helped by considering what would happen if we did not have risk assessments.

## ✎ Learner answer

Risk assessment is important. If we did not assess risks, many more accidents would happen. Employers must make the workplace safe, ensure machinery is safe and that safe systems of work are set and followed. They must make sure articles and substances are moved, stored and used safely, provide adequate welfare facilities, train workers on health and safety and consult workers on these matters.

Part of making a workplace safe and having safe systems of work includes conducting a risk assessment. An activities coordinator organising a trip to a local garden centre must risk assess the situation. The people going on the trip have differing mobility needs. One person uses a wheelchair. One uses a walking stick. Several are slow walkers and tire easily. There are many hazards.

The coach must be able to accommodate wheelchair users and those with poor mobility or they may fall trying to get on the coach **(a)**. Seatbelts must be available and worn. If people do not wear seatbelts they may be severely injured if there was an accident **(a)**. If the coach is not safe, an accident may occur **(a)**. The driver must be safe and have had sufficient rest before driving, or he may cause an accident **(b)**.

On arrival, there may be hazards at the garden centre. Wet floors and congested areas are hazards for those with poor mobility. People may slip, trip or fall **(a)**. A wheelchair user needs space to move round. Most garden centres are aware of this but the activities coordinator should check the place before the visit to make sure it is safe **(b)**.

Sometimes people can get lost in a strange place **(a)**, so there should be a pre-arranged meeting place and time that everyone knows, such as the café **(b)**. Those who tire easily can rest while they wait. It is also important to make sure everyone knows where the toilets are and that toilets for wheelchair users are available to avoid distress **(b)**.

There should be a contact back at base and a minimum of two staff on the trip. If one of the residents becomes ill and has to go to hospital there will still be a member of staff to look after the rest **(b)**.

By following the five-step process, accidents can be avoided:

1. Identify the hazards
2. Decide who might be harmed and how
3. Evaluate the risks and decide on precautions
4. Record your findings and implement them
5. Review your assessment and update if necessary.

**Assessor report:** The learner has made a good start in explaining the importance of assessing risks.

## Assessor report – overall

*What is good about this assessment evidence?*

The learner has thought through possible hazards, explained what might happen if things go wrong **(a)** and how to avoid accidents **(b)**.

*What could be improved about this assessment evidence?*

Although the learner has mentioned employer responsibilities, they have not yet mentioned the Health and Safety at Work Act 1974. This should be included. It would be good to mention that health and safety is the responsibility of everyone, not just the employee.

## (2B.D2) Evaluate the importance of the use of risk assessments in health and social care, using selected examples

Assessor report: The command verb in the grading criteria is **evaluate**. In the learner's answer we would expect to see a considered judgement on the importance of risk assessments in health and social care. This should be based on detailed information about the use of risk assessments to maximise the safety of service users. These examples could be brought forward from 2B.M2 if they are sufficiently detailed.

### ✎ Learner answer

Risk assessment does not eliminate risk; it manages risk. There may at times be a conflict between the service user's right to take risks and the employer's responsibility to provide a safe environment. For example, a day trip to the seaside for people with learning disabilities will help them gain confidence and develop a social network, but they may run the risk of meeting prejudice from the public.

Risk assessments reduce the risk of harm. They do not get rid of hazards but instead help us to manage the hazard so no one suffers injury.

If we did not have risk assessments, accidents would happen much more often. People would suffer harm and may even die. If we did not do a risk assessment for a trip to a garden centre **(a)**, someone could fall trying to get onto a coach with high steps, or someone could get hurt as they try to carry a wheelchair up the coach steps. At the garden centre, people could slip on wet floors or trip over pot plants on the floor, and potentially fracture their hip.

Without a prearranged meeting place, someone could get lost or be left behind when the others go home. If the driver and coach were not safe there might be an accident and people could get killed.

In evaluating their importance , we have only to look at what might happen if we do not use them. They are vitally important to reduce risk and prevent harm to staff, residents, and visitors, in fact to everyone **(b)**.

**Assessor report:** The learner has made a good start in evaluating the importance of risk assessments.

## Assessor report – overall

### What is good about this assessment evidence?

The learner gives detail from a specific situation **(a)** to support their argument for the importance of risk assessments. They draw together their argument and make an evaluative statement **(b)**.

### What could be improved about this assessment evidence?

2B.D2 requires selected examples; therefore more than one example is needed. It would be good practice to give two other examples to support the evaluation.

## 2B.P4 Describe how the right to confidentiality is protected in health and social care

Assessor report: The command verb in the grading criteria is **describe**. In the learner's answer we would expect to see a detailed description of how confidentiality is protected in health and social care.

### ✍ Learner answer

> Confidentiality – keeping information private – is important in health and social care because service users give a lot of personal information to care professionals and do not expect that information to be discussed with non-professionals.

Assessor report: The learner has made a good start in describing *why* confidentiality is important in health and social care. They now need to describe *how* the right to confidentiality is protected.

### ✍ Learner answer

> There are several ways that the right to confidentiality is protected. All records must be accurate and factual. Paper-based records should be dated and signed **(a)**. If they are on a computer they must be protected by a password and an individual log-in that shows who has made the record and when it was made **(b)**.
>
> All records must be stored safely and not left where members of the public can see them. Information on computer screens should not be visible to people waiting at a health centre reception desk **(b)**. Paper-based records should be stored in the manager's office in a care home, or in a central office in a day centre **(a)**. Computer-held records in hospitals, health centres, care homes and social work offices must be backed up and stored under password protection **(b)**.
>
> Information should only be retrieved by authorised people. No one should give their password to others to get electronic information **(b)**. Notes should not be left at the end of the bed in hospital, where anyone can pick them up and read them **(a)**.

**Assessor report:** The learner has made a good start in describing how the right to confidentiality is protected in health and social care.

## Assessor report – overall

**What is good about this assessment evidence?**

The learner has considered paper-based **(a)** and electronic records **(b)** and has used examples from different settings.

**What could be improved about this assessment evidence?**

The learner should also consider how confidentiality is protected with transmitting verbal information and also with photographs, mobile phones and social media.

**Explain why the right to confidentiality is protected in health and social care, using examples**

**Assessor report:** The command verb in the grading criteria is explain. In the learner's answer we would expect to see a detailed explanation of why the right to confidentiality is protected in health and social care, using examples which can be from case studies or from the news. The learner should refer to data protection legislation to show the right of service users to confidentiality. Sections of the Human Rights Act may also be useful.

✎ **Learner answer**

The Data Protection Act 1998 applies to all forms of media, including paper and electronic, and covers holding, obtaining, recording, using and disclosing of information that identifies living individuals **(a)**.

It is important to protect the right to confidentiality so that no one is harmed. Service users trust professionals to keep information secure. If care professionals break that confidentiality then service users may no longer trust them and may stop using the services. Breaking that confidentiality may cause harm to that person **(b)**.

**Assessor report:** The learner has made a good start in explaining why the right to confidentiality is protected in health and social care. They now need to refer to relevant examples.

✎ **Learner answer**

Here is an example that shows why the right to confidentiality is protected in health and social care. A nurse was reviewing Mr X's paper-based care plan with him in a side room. She checked the details to make sure he was the correct Mr X, and went through the treatment he had so far for his HIV positive status. She did the review in a side room to ensure privacy. Unfortunately, during the review she was called away to deal with an urgent telephone call. She apologised to Mr X and explained they would continue the review later. She took the notes with her and put them in the notes trolley in the office before answering the phone call. Mr X appreciated her thorough approach to storing his records safely and to keeping his health issues confidential. He is worried that if his boss knows he is HIV positive they will find an excuse to sack him **(c)**.

Under the Data Protection Act 1998 medical information should be kept secure. It should be relevant and up to date and the patient must be allowed to see what is written about them if they request to do so. It should not be disclosed to those who do not need to know **(a)**.

**Assessor report:** The learner has made a good start in evaluating the importance of risk assessments.

## Assessor report – overall

**What is good about this assessment evidence?**

The learner refers to legislation **(a)**, says why it is important to protect the right to confidentiality **(b)** and gives a case study to show how this works in practice **(c)**.

**What could be improved about this assessment evidence?**

Examples are required; therefore the learner should provide more than one. It would be good to see examples from a range of settings. The learner's case study refers to paper-based records only; it would be good to include a case study that includes electronically held records and their recording, storage and transmission could be used to further explain why the right to confidentiality is protected in health and social care. Sections of the Human Rights Act could also be referred to.

## 2B.D3 Justify occasions where there is a need for an employee to breach confidentiality, using examples

**Assessor report:** The command verb in the grading criteria is **justify**. In the learner's answer we would expect to see reasons for when confidentiality can be breached by employees. This should be supported by examples.

### ✍ Learner answer

> Confidentiality is important but sometimes it is important to break confidentiality to safeguard other individuals, to safeguard a service user, or to report criminal activities.
>
> Janie, a 20-year-old girl with learning difficulties, lives in supported accommodation. One of the day staff, Tom, finds Janie crying in her room. Janie tells Tom that she has no money left because the other residents in the house make her give them her money so they can buy cigarettes. She does not want anyone to know in case they bully her. Tom gently explains that in order to protect her he will have to tell his line manager so they can work out how to keep her safe from bullying. She is a vulnerable person because she has learning disabilities, and the carer's duty is to safeguard service users.

**Assessor report:** The learner has made a good start by justifying an occasion when it is necessary to breach confidentiality to protect a vulnerable service user.

### Assessor report – overall

**What is good about this assessment evidence?**

The learner has given a realistic situation where financial and emotional abuse justify breaching confidentiality.

**What could be improved about this assessment evidence?**

At least two more examples are required to achieve 2B.D3. It would be good to see a range of examples from different sectors of health and social care. Examples could be drawn from the media or from case studies.

# Sample assignment brief 1: Investigate the rights of individuals using health and social care services

## Learning aim A

| ASSIGNMENT TITLE | The rights of individuals using health and social care services |
|---|---|
| LEARNING AIM | 2A |
| CRITERIA COVERED | 2A.P1, 2A.P2, ,2A.M1, 2A.D1 |
| ASSESSMENT EVIDENCE | Handwritten or word-processed notebook |

This assignment will assess the following learning aim and grading criteria:

**Learning aim A:** Investigate the rights of individuals using health and social care services.

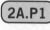 Summarise the individual rights of service users in health and social care.

 Describe how current and relevant legislation protects the rights of service users, using examples.

 Explain ways in which service users' individual rights can be upheld in health and social care, using selected examples.

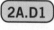 Assess the benefits and potential difficulties of upholding service users' rights in health and social care, using selected examples.

## Scenario

You are considering a career in health and social work and are about to start a voluntary placement to find out if this career would suit you. Before starting you want to find out as much as you can about the rights of people who use health and social care services. You gather information into a notebook to help you when you start.

# Task 1

Write a short review of the rights of individuals in health and social care. Briefly explain each of these rights: to be respected; to be treated as an individual; to be treated with dignity; to be treated equally and not discriminated against; to be allowed privacy and confidentiality; to be allowed access to information about self; to have account taken of their own choices; to be allowed independence; to be safe; to able to take risks; and to be involved in their own care.

# Task 2

Describe how current and relevant legislation protects the rights of service users, including the Equality Act (2010). Describe at least two ways that legislation protects the rights of service users and apply this to a group of service users such as patients in hospital or residents in a care home.

# Task 3

Give details of how to uphold service users' individual rights using examples from health and social care. You will need three detailed examples from a range of health and social care settings to show the ways rights can be upheld. Refer to the legislation that gives these rights.

# Task 4

Assess the benefits to upholding service users' rights which will help service users and staff. There are also difficulties in doing this. Difficulties may happen when service users' rights conflict, when both have rights which affect others. There are also difficulties in upholding rights when they conflict with the responsibilities of staff. For this section you need to say what the benefits are and what the difficulties are, using examples from health and social care to illustrate what you mean. Try to come to a conclusion as to whether or not the benefits outweigh the difficulties.

# Sample assignment brief 2: Examine the responsibilities of employers and employees

## Learning aim B

| ASSIGNMENT TITLE | The responsibilities of employers and employees in upholding service users' rights in health and social care |
|---|---|
| LEARNING AIM | 2B |
| CRITERIA COVERED | 2B.P3, 2B.M2, 2B.D2, 2B.P4, 2B.M3, 2B.D3 |
| ASSESSMENT EVIDENCE | Handwritten or word-processed notebook |

This assignment will assess the following learning aim and grading criteria:

**Learning aim B:** Examine the responsibilities of employers and employees.

 **2B.P3** Describe how an employee can plan to maximise the safety of service users.

 **2B.M2** Explain why risk assessment is important in health and social care.

**2B.D2** Evaluate the importance of the use of risk assessments in health and social care, using selected examples.

 **2B.P4** Describe how the right to confidentiality is protected in health and social care.

 **2B.M3** Explain why the right to confidentiality is protected in health and social care, using examples.

**2B.D3** Justify occasions where there is a need for an employee to breach confidentiality, using examples.

## Scenario

You are considering a career in health and social work and are about to start a voluntary placement to find out if this career would suit you. Before starting you want to find out as much as you can about the responsibilities that employers and employees have in making sure that service users have their rights. You gather information into a notebook to help you when you start.

## Task 1

Describe the main ways an employee can make the service users as safe as possible in a specific health and social care setting. Look at risk assessment, safeguarding, and other ways, such as control of substances harmful to health, the use of protective equipment, infection control, reporting and recording accidents and incidents, dealing with complaints, the provision of staff toilets, washing facilities and drinking water, and the provision of first aid facilities.

## Task 2

Explain why risk assessment is important in health and soical care. Focus on a specific situation, such as planning a trip to the local theatre for residents of a care home, or a shopping trip for a small group of people with learning disabilities. Refer to legislation such as the Health and Safety at Work Act 1974, and give a detailed explanation of the importance of risk assessment in the situation.

## Task 3

Based on information about the use of risk assessments, weigh up the evidence for and against the importance of risk assessments in health and social care. Decide how important risk assessments are, based on the evidence you present. These examples could be brought forward from Task 2 if they are sufficiently detailed.

## Task 4

Using examples, give a detailed description of how confidentiality is protected in health and social care. This should include the recording, storing and retrieval of paper-based and electronic records. It should also include how to maintain confidentiality when giving information verbally.

## Task 5

Give a detailed explanation of why the right to confidentiality is protected in health and social care, using examples from case studies or from the news. Refer to data protection legislation to show why it is important to protect the right to confidentiality. You may also find sections of the Human Rights Act are useful too.

## Task 6

Give valid reasons for when confidentiality can be breached by employees. These should be supported by examples from health and social care. You may wish to use case studies from the news to support your case.

# Assessment criteria

| Level 2 Pass | Level 2 Merit | Level 2 Distinction |
|---|---|---|
| Learning aim A: Investigate the rights of individuals using health and social care services | | |
| 2A.P1 Summarise the individual rights of service users in health and social care. | 2A.M1 Explain ways in which service users' individual rights can be upheld in health and social care, using selected examples. | 2A.D1 Assess the benefits and potential difficulties of upholding service users' rights in health and social care, using selected examples. |
| 2A.P2 Describe how current and relevant legislation protects the rights of service users, using examples. | | |
| Learning aim B: Examine the responsibilities of employers and employees in upholding service users' rights in health and social care | | |
| 2B.P3 Describe how an employee can plan to maximise the safety of service users. | 2B.M2 Explain why risk assessment is important in health and social care. | 2B.D2 Evaluate the importance of the use of risk assessments in health and social care, using selected examples. |
| 2B.P4 Describe how the right to confidentiality is protected in health and social care. | 2B.M3 Explain why the right to confidentiality is protected in health and social care, using examples. | 2B.D3 Justify occasions where there is a need for an employee to breach confidentiality, using examples. |

# Knowledge recap answers

## Learning aim A: Investigate the rights of individuals using health and social care services

1. Eleven rights of individuals using health and social care services:
   - to be respected
   - be treated as an individual
   - to be treated with dignity
   - to be treated equally and not discriminated against
   - to be allowed privacy and confidentiality
   - to be allowed access to information about self
   - to have account taken of own choices, e.g. to communicate in preferred method/language
   - to be allowed independence
   - to be safe
   - to be able to take risks
   - to be involved in own care.

2. Three examples of legislation that protect the rights of service users:
   - Human Rights Act (1998)
   - Equality Act (2010)
   - Mental Health Act (1983) revised 2007.

3. Five ways that care workers can uphold the rights of service users:
   - anti-discriminatory practices
   - ensuring privacy during personal care
   - offering a person-centred approach
   - showing empathy
   - being honest.

## Learning aim B: Examine the responsibilities of employers and employees in upholding service users' rights in health and social care

1. Employers and the people who work for them, the employees, must ensure the safety of service users.

2. The five steps in risk assessment are:
   - Identify the hazards
   - Decide who might be harmed and how
   - Evaluate the risks and decide on precautions
   - Record your findings and implement them
   - Review your assessment and update if necessary.

3. A *hazard* is anything that may cause harm, such as loose carpet, wet floor or trailing cord. A *risk* is the chance, high or low, that somebody could be harmed by these and other hazards, together with an indication of how serious the harm could be.

4. Breaches of confidentiality are appropriate to safeguard other individual(s); to safeguard a service user; or to report criminal activities.

5. Any two laws relating to confidentiality from: The Data Protection Act 1998; The Freedom of Information Act 2000; The Police and Criminal Evidence Act 1984.

# Index

Index